1

A Matter of Life and Health

What is Keeping You from Being Fit
and How You Can Beat It!

By Bob Flynn

Title: A Matter of Life and Health
Subtitle: What is Keeping You from Being Fit
and How You Can Beat It!
Bob Flynn
Published by: Bob Flynn

ISBN: 9781090200952

First Edition, 2019
Published in U.S.A.

I dedicate this book to my wife Tricia, and three children Christian, Matthew, and Meagan for helping me unconditionally through this amazing journey.

Disclaimer

This book is designed to provide information on ideas for a healthy lifestyle only. This information is provided and sold with the knowledge that the publisher and author do not offer any legal, medical, or other professional advice. In the case of a need for any such expertise consult with the appropriate professional. This book does not contain all information available on the subject. This book has not been created to be specific to any individual's or organizations' situation or needs. Every effort has been made to make this book as accurate as possible. However, there may be typographical and or content errors. Therefore, this book should serve only as a general guide and not as the ultimate source of subject information. This book contains information that might be dated and is intended only to educate and entertain. The author and publisher shall have no liability or responsibility to any person or entity regarding any loss or damage incurred, or alleged to have incurred, directly or indirectly, by the information contained in this book.

Table of Contents

Introduction

After owning a thriving health club for a decade, and despite working out on average 3 days a week with a personal trainer at high intensity, most of the time I barely had the energy to be a couch potato. What energy I did have was used to make my way from the couch to the refrigerator and I was still hungry all the time.

My weight was 245 lbs., body fat percentage of was 26.1 and visceral fat rating was 13. All considered to be in the overfat range. No wonder I did not have any energy. The weight and body fat I was carrying around, even though I am considered tall at 6'-3", put me into the danger zone for a whole host of risky diseases at 53 years old.

Because I had an appetite all the time, my second helpings could have taken first place in the buffet line. Not only was my calorie intake out of control my food choices were not the best.

Then at my annual physical I boasted to my Doctor about my dedication to working out regularly. He asked, "How do you feel?" I had to admit I was sadly lacking in the energy department.

After a few tests and results I got some disheartening news. My BMI was 32 and cholesterol levels were over 300. My doctor said, "No wonder you are tired," and gave me a healthy eating brochure. I was at high risk for problems and have a genetic history of heart disease.

This was a 'wake up' call and I decided to answer. After all I was 'sick and tired of being tired' and did not want to leave my fantastic wife (married 28 years) and three wonderful grown children by going out early if I could prevent it.

Here I am today...

I am at my goal weight with so much energy I travel the country to participate in triathlons at 53 years old. *And I feel great!*

I want the same for you... living at your ideal weight, having all the energy you need, and add years to your life. So, I became a health coach and am sharing my story, discoveries and guidance with you in this book.

This is my mission for you; a life of zest.

This book is a heart to heart talk between you and me about improving your health, your life and reaching your goals.

Bob Flynn
MissionZest.com

1. Why Is This Not Your Fault?

Today, more than 60% of Americans are so overweight they are in the obese category. This is about 100 million people and the numbers are growing. The child obesity rate has doubled in the last two decades.

Obesity leads to discrimination in public, school, the workplace and social settings. Insurance premiums often increase and can be policies can be canceled. Being overweight can sap your energy, cause discomfort, attack self-esteem, wreck relationships, limit activities, lead to disability and be fatal. Being overweight is dangerous with a host of health issues and diseases that have a direct correlation.

If you have ever battled weight control, struggled to be fit, or suffered any health issues due to diet or being overweight *I have news for you.*

This is not your fault.

In fact, if you feel losing weight and staying at your ideal weight is almost impossible, and a constant battle... the truth is there are some giants working very hard against you.

Thousands of companies are spending billions of dollars to keep you from being healthy. These corporations include food producers, food distributors, advertising agencies, grocery stores, fast food, the pharmaceutical industry and even the credit card companies.

They are not necessarily evil. However, these giants of the food industry are doing a great job promoting their products and many hinder the health of an entire population.

How are Giants Working Feverishly and Spending Billions of Dollars to Keep You from Being Healthy?

The food industry and associated companies have a myriad of manipulative, sly, and downright deceitful tactics and methods in their arsenal for product creation, packaging, advertising, displaying and marketing. However, before we tar and feather these corporations be aware that not all these tactics were created at one time or to inevitably deceive or defraud the public and some companies are more involved (guilty) than others. Such is the game of capitalism and government attempts at regulation. Knowing all this occurs will only benefit you when you understand how the methods work and what you can do to personally combat these tactics and protect your health.

Manipulation occurs by marketing to instant gratification, creating edible substances that satisfy taste with little or no focus on nutrition, developing brands that obscure nutritional value and even identity, and exploiting the five food disconnects.

Marketing to Instant Gratification

"The obsession with instant gratification blinds us from our long-term potential."
- Mike Dooley

Who doesn't *'want it now'?*

The massive credit card industry has capitalized on our desires for instant gratification, and so has the food industry. The convenience of speed and satisfying instant gratification has fueled the fast food business that boast chains with thousands of locations. Regrettably, in most cases we are sacrificing healthy nutrition for a quick fix.

Due to the delay for the brain to acknowledge our food intake, we often eat fast and more than we should. Then when we get undesirable results in the forms of excess weight and being out of shape, we seek instant gratification to correct our situation with fad diets, supplement or diet drinks, and pills.

One reason that diets seldom work is that they require something in direct conflict with instant gratification; denial. Losing weight and getting fit also requires time as well as effort and commitment.

Store shelves are stacked with processed foods that aim to satisfy with instant gratification. Foods that can be eaten with little or no preparation.

The choices for fast and prepared foods is dizzying. The National Restaurant Association, reports that annual restaurant sales are more than over five hundred billion dollars and there are more than one million restaurants in the U.S.

Another example is one of my favorite foods; pizza. This industry has been growing by leaps and bounds. Americans eat an average of 23 pounds of pizza per year! Sadly, pizza is loaded with fat burdened cheeses on a foundation of not so healthy dough.

What are the Five Food Disconnects That Can Keep You from Being Healthy?

I am about to reveal to you what is preventing most people from living a healthy life at their desired weight and with the energy they deserve.

Yes! You deserve to live at your ideal weight with all the energy you need, sleep well, and feel good!

- So, what is making people obese and why is all the dieting in the world not helping them reach and maintain a healthy weight?
- Why are more people reporting that they are chronically tired than ever before?

The answer:
Our relationship with food is broken.

What has so damaged our relationship with food?

The answer:
There are 5 Food Disconnects raising havoc with our health and wrecking our weight.

1. The Identification Disconnect

We often have no idea how many calories we are eating or even what we are eating.

Just a century or so ago, the greater number of people were eating from their farms or local farms and consuming mostly whole foods. People prepared most all their meals and there were only a few processed foods available. This was part of a slower life pace that gave people a relationship with their nourishment.

Today, few people grow their own food and planning meals, grocery shopping, preparing food, and cleaning up meals at home is time people would prefer spending other ways. People want food that is ready to eat or easily prepared such as microwavable. All you need to do is take a stroll around your local grocery stores to see how easy to prepare or ready to eat processed foods dominate the shelf space. As far as the number of items available, whole foods are frequently less than ten per cent of all items. There is no argument that whole foods and specifically organic meats, produce, and dairy are healthier choices than processes foods.

[1]Yet according to the American Institute for Cancer Research if you're like the average American, more than half of your diet is filled with processed foods.

They cite a study that found that for the average America:

- more than one-half of calories came from ultra-processed foods

---

[1] http://blog.aicr.org/2017/06/13/processed-foods-calories-and-nutrients-americans-alarming-diet/

- less than one-third of calories were from unprocessed or minimally processed foods
- about 12 percent of calories came from the other foods' category.

The more ultra-processed foods you eat, the less protein, fiber, vitamins A, C, D and E, potassium and calcium you get. And you consume more added sugars, saturated fat and overall carbohydrates in their diets.

In addition, processed foods and capitalism marketing have contributed to the American disconnection with food. There are thousands of processed food names that eradicate any chance of depicting the actual ingredients.

Here are some popular American processed foods and drinks you might recognize but can you name the ingredients?

Apple Jacks
Cheerios
Bugles

Special K
Grape Nuts
Hamburger Helper
Happy Meal
Snapple
Jelly Bellies
Animal Crackers
Fruit Loops
Frosted Flakes
Twinkies
Boo Berry
Total
Captain Crunch
Lucky Charms
Chex
Pop Secret
Big Mac
Whopper
Nestle's Quick
Pepsi
Dr. Pepper
Haagen-Dazs
Aunt Jemima

Eggo
Pop Tarts
Pizza Rolls
Doritos
Hungry Jack
Peter Pan
Chips Ahoy
Teddy Grahams
Goldfish
Butterfinger
Milky Way
Snickers
Gatorade

There are many more. These are products that most Americans recognize and grew up knowing. But imagine if you lived 150 years ago and could time travel to today. By the product name, you would not know what is in any one of these foods.

For example, did you know there are no grapes, or any part of a grape, or any nuts in

'Grape Nuts'? If you have been a fan of Grape Nuts, I am sorry to 'crush your grape'!

Quick, how many of the 27 ingredients in a Twinkie can you name?

If you said water, flour, salt, or sugar you are right. But that still leaves over 20 other ingredients.

While twinkies might not be a staple of your diet, they have been a prized dessert or snack for kids for decades (and they are still popular).

The Good (and there is very little): Twinkies do tout 20 mg of calcium each, yet they do not provide a significant amount of any other vitamins, minerals or nutrients.

The Bad: In addition to a myriad of risky ingredients, one Twinkie contains 19 grams of sugar or almost five teaspoons. [2]The American Heart Association recommends keeping added

---

[2] https://www.livestrong.com/article/310643-twinkies-nutrition/

sugar intake to six teaspoons per day for women and nine teaspoons per day for men.

2. The Preparation Disconnect

[3]We no longer prepare our food like we once did. The ready-to-eat pasta company Artisola commissioned its State of Home Cooking Survey, which found that only 27 percent of Americans cook a meal every day.

When you do not prepare your own food, you often have no idea what the ingredients are. In addition, when you eat out or get take out, you no longer control your portions.

3. The Dining Disconnect

Even when we sit down to finally relax and eat, many of our meals no longer focus on the food. We have business lunches, dinner dates, and breakfast meetings. We gather to eat for

---

3 https://wtop.com/food-restaurant/2018/03/only-27-percent-of-americans-cook-every-day-survey-says/

celebrations of anniversaries, birthdays, reunions, promotions, etc.

Just visit any lunch crowd and count how many people are on their cell phones while eating.

We often mix entertainment with food. We watch movies, series, and sports all while eating. Often the choices include pizza, fast food, chips, and other less than nutritious snacks and meals.

4. The Origin Disconnect

While we have an unprecedented array of food choices, we no longer associate with our food's origins. With world trade many of our foods and ingredients derive from countries across the globe. Some of these countries have far fewer health standards for farming and water purity.

5. The Health Correlation Disconnect

Processed foods have gained acceptance even with confusing and unfamiliar ingredients and origins unknown to us. Most of society has no idea what they are putting into their bodies daily.

2. What Can You Do About Nutrition and Eating?

"Let food be thy medicine and medicine be thy food." - Hippocrates

What are Meal Plans and How Can They Help You?

Meal plans are schedules you make about what you are going to eat for the week. This could include beautiful presentations, 21 individual meals where breakfast, lunch, and dinner are all decided, and perfect macronutrient ratios so that you optimize your health. Or meal planning could mean 3 dinners that you are dedicated to making at home each week.

Why Meal Plans?

Meal plans enable you to eat right while you save time, money, and energy. By preparing ahead of time you can reduce stress around dinner and make healthier choices.

Save Time

How much time have you wasted standing in front of the refrigerator trying to decide what to eat only to choose the same old thing? Knowing what you are going to eat reduces time wasted in indecision and cuts down on last minute trips to the grocery store.

Save Money with Meal Plans

Using your groceries efficiently will reduce the cost of shopping. Instead of letting spinach go bad in the fridge each week, use up what you have before shopping for more. Eating at home will save you a pretty penny as the cost is roughly half that of eating out.

Eat Healthy

We make poorer decisions when we are tired or hungry. By being deliberate about our shopping and cooking, we can cut down on the pull to eat high-calorie, low-nutrient food.

Control Portions

Meal plans make overeating harder. By allocating a certain amount of food to each meal, you make eating more calories less attractive.

Reduce Stress with Meal Plans

Most of us have hectic lives and seem to just squeeze in enough time to eat. We have anxiety about our unhealthy diets–which creates more stress because we aren't giving our bodies what they need. In the short run, a meal plan eases tension about what to eat in the morning; in the long run, making health a priority will reduce overall stress.

Tailor meal plans to your specific schedule and dietary needs. You can become healthier and more energized with reduced effort if you put in a bit of forethought.

Meal Planning for Weight Loss
Meal planning for weight loss helps you reach your goals by making the best options easily

available. Losing weight can be difficult but if you prep and plan your meals and snacks before you are hungry, you are more likely to make better choices.

What Should You Do When Meal Planning for Weight Loss?

Eat lots of protein

Aim for 30% of your calories to be protein. Protein makes you feel full by triggering the production of ghrelin, the "satiety hormone." When you feel full, you eat less. Start your day with healthy proteins like nuts and seeds, Greek yogurt, beans, eggs, or chicken breast.

Portion your snacks

Portion control is an important aspect of weight loss. Pack ½ to 1 cup servings of low-carb vegetables like broccoli, tomatoes, radishes, asparagus, and cucumbers into small Tupperware containers or sandwich bags. Meal planning for weight loss allows you to grab healthy snacks on-the-go instead of choosing fast food or a granola bar.

Eat lots of soluble fiber

Soluble fiber forms a gel in your stomach by absorbing water. This substance slows down the release of food into your gut which keeps you feeling fuller, longer. Oatmeal, apples, beans, potatoes, and whole grains contain a lot of soluble fiber.

Stock up on greens

When meal planning for weight loss, eat food that has low energy density. You get the sensation of being full, from the volume of food that you eat, not the calories. You want to eat as few calories as possible while filling you up. Raw spinach, kale, and swiss chard are all nutrient dense and low calorie, making them a great choice when meal planning for weight loss.

What Should You Avoid When Meal Planning for Weight Loss?

Most low-fat products are high in sugar. Try to focus on eating healthy fats. Monounsaturated fats like in avocados, nuts, and olive oil; and polyunsaturated fats like in fish, flax, and chia seeds are part of a healthy diet.

Empty your pantry

One of the surest ways to gain weight is to make high sugar, highly processed food easily available. Go through your fridge, freezer, and pantry and throw out anything that you want to avoid eating when meal planning for weight loss.

Meal planning for weight loss with be easy if you follow these few tips. Consider downloading a calorie counting app like MyFitnessPal or Noom to help you reach your goals.

How Minerals and Nutrients Help Muscles

How do minerals and nutrients help muscles? How confusing it is for the average health vs non-health conscious individual to make good choices on improving their eating. Beliefs that gluten free is a better choice than gluten products even if you not gluten sensitive/or have Celiac's Disease. Also, Sugar. What is high fructose corn syrup and why is it something you need to look for in your product choices. Butter vs. Margarine. The need for healthy fats. I'm sure you get the idea.

We need to look at the body as a whole to make sure our patients/clients focused on their total well-being in order to heal well. Water intake for hydration, calcium intake, sodium intake, etc. All the muscles in the body from your heart, brain and limb moving muscles work better with necessary minerals and nutrients.

Minerals and Nutrients Help Muscles

What do you need to make your body work best? You need micronutrients and macronutrients. Simply put vitamins and minerals are called micronutrients because the body needs them in smaller amounts than macronutrients also known as carbohydrates, proteins, and fats. Vitamins and minerals do not provide energy (calories), but they help to release energy from the macros. Overall, there are 13 essential vitamins: vitamins A, C, D, E, K, and 8 B vitamins and they benefit your eyes, skin, cell growth, bones, blood and reproduction.

There are 16 essential minerals: calcium, phosphorus, potassium, sulfur, sodium, chloride, magnesium, iron, zinc, copper, manganese, iodine, and selenium, molybdenum, chromium, and fluoride. These minerals are important for energy production, blood pressure, immune health, bone and tooth health, fluid and electrolyte balance, and muscle and nerve function. By eating a variety of nutrient-dense foods from the 5 food groups, you will have a mineral-rich and vitamin-rich diet.

Minerals are best supplied to your body by ingesting specific foods rich with the mineral (e.g., calcium in milk) or added to the food (e.g., orange juice with added calcium; iodized salt fortified with iodine). Diet can meet all the body's requirements, although supplements can be used when some requirements (e.g., calcium) are not adequately met through ones eating style, or when deficiencies arise from illness, injury, etc. There are many uses for supplements, but it is best to have your diet assessed in order to be made aware of what your body may be lacking in order to maintain optimal health. Now you know how minerals and nutrients help muscles.

3. How Can You Instill Positive Behavior Change Once and For All?

"A habit is something you can do without thinking - which is why most of us have so many of them."
- Frank A. Clark

Have you ever thought about how all your current habits began? The fact is most if not all of our habits are not intentional. When we diagnose how our habits started, we realize they were usually not well thought out plans.

For example, for many years as an adult I had pancakes, bacon and eggs for breakfast every morning. Not until I evaluated my habits, did I realize my menu choices were the same breakfast Mom made every morning before school.

For many years I had a habit of putting gas in my car only when the big 'E' for EMPTY on the gauge was tempting the needle. I even ran out of gas once or twice. Only when I was considering the sources of all my habits did I realize this habit was rooted in my teenage years when I began driving my first car. I was always scrounging for gas money and often running on fumes.

One of my coaching subjects, Heather, told me how much she hated shopping. Even though she made a list of healthy foods, her anxiety at the store led to some poor food choices.

When I asked several questions about her shopping, like where she shops, what she does not like, etc. she finally said, "I do not like crowds."

"When do you shop?" I inquired.

"Saturday morning," she answered.

"Why?" I asked.

"Because that is when I have always shopped. I work during the week," Heather responded.

After some discussion we discovered her average time in the store each week was about 30 minutes, she works just up the street from where she shops, and she gets one hour for lunch every week day.

I suggested she try shopping on her lunch hour every Friday.

A few weeks later Heather exclaimed, "I love grocery shopping again! There are far less people in the store, the anxiety is gone, and I focus on buying only what is on my list."

Yes, something so simple, got Heather on a healthier diet. We often cannot see the forest for the trees when it comes to our behaviors and habits.

Heather's habit of making a list of healthy foods to buy and grocery shopping once a week did not change. Only the *when* changed in this instance.

This is important because when we evaluate our habits, their derivatives, and ask the who, what, when, why, and how for each one, we often discover the habit might not need be eliminated but altered.

In fact, altering even the worst habits to change the behavior can have better results. For example, if you sit and like to watch the news or your favorite show every day for a half hour or so, don't stop watching. Just watch while you walk on a treadmill or ride a stationary bicycle. This one behavior adjustment could get you fit, happy with your body and health, and extend your life.

I did not stop my habit of eating breakfast at the same time each day. I altered what is on my plate.

Altering your old habits and replacing them with new healthy habits will help you reach your nutrition goals.

Create S.M.A.R.T. Goals

Setting unrealistic goals is setting yourself up for failure. Vague objectives give you no place to end and no way to celebrate successes.

SMART stands for

- Specific
- Measurable
- Attainable
- Realistic
- Timely

Setting goals gives you what to aim for and setting SMART goals helps you achieve them.

A health coach can help. In my program I first do a comprehensive evaluation of where you are with weight, sleep, nutrition, exercise, and any concerns. Then I can help you set specific and realistic goals within a time period that makes your goals attainable. We establish measurable progress data points that track your progress throughout your journey, and I recommend timely adjustments as needed.

But there is far more to getting and staying fit than just goals. We need to evaluate and maintain your attitude of optimism and keep you accountable and motivated.

Motivation

If you want to get fit but struggle to stay motivated, you are hardly alone. Over 160 million Americans are overweight or obese. Here are a few ways to get and stay on the right track:

Find an Accountability Partner

Finding an accountability partner is a way to leverage peer pressure in your favor. One study found that committing to a specific goal with someone increases your chances of achieving that goal by 65%. Reach out to your support network or an online community to find someone you can depend on.

Get A Health Coach to Stay Motivated

An accountability partner functions well because you make a social commitment to a goal. A health coach pairs that same accountability with loss aversion "losses loom larger than gains" and while the motivation to stay fit may wane, motivation to make your money work for you will stay strong.

Focus on The Feeling

How do you stay motivated once you have reached your weight or measurement goals? By taking pride and feeling joy in the process. People who eat well and exercise often report higher levels of energy and well-being. Pay attention to subtle improvements in your mood.

Be Clear on Your Reasons

Get clarity on why your health is a priority. Fitness is an end goal for some people but many of us find more meaning in another area of life—our children, grandchildren, or self-esteem.

Find Exercise and Food You Enjoy

Nothing will zap you of motivation than food that makes you gag and exercise that makes you feel weak. Find what works for you. Preparing meals with friends is a great way to explore the culinary world and walking with a dog may put a bounce in your step.

Finding your 'why' and a regiment that works for you may take some time and tinkering but the extra effort will allow success to come easier. Your 'why' is the reason or list of reasons that you want to be fit. You want to get to your root 'why.'

For example, if you want to get in shape to fit into your old jeans and attract a mate, your chances of maintaining fitness are less. Getting fit for appearance reasons to attract a mate might work in the short run, but once you land a partner, your work has paid off. You will need to find a new why.

Fitness is a long-term goal that requires ongoing motivation to energize you from one step to the next, week after week.

You only have one body and you want your health to last for your life so that you can enjoy every minute and live as long you can.

Depravity

A frequent error when making nutritional and eating habit changes is the perception of sacrificing. This perception is often associated with diets and dieting.

When you deny yourself usual pleasures such as from junk food or alcohol and see denying these habits as sacrifices, you will struggle to stay on track. Then when you do reach your goals you might see indulging in old habits as rewarding. This makes the potential of making long-term changes stick less likely.

If you ever have dieted by elimination of certain foods such as cutting down on carbs and ruling out bread and pasta, you focus on what you are missing. This can trigger reward, deserve, and rebellion reactions.

'I deserve just a slice of bread,'

'I have not had bread in a week. Some will not hurt me now.'

You might resort to the rebellion reaction telling yourself: 'I can eat what I want. I have power over food and after all I have demonstrated this for a week now.'

In order to avoid these drawbacks, start with a mindset of choice:

'I can eat whatever I want, though I am choosing health over being unhealthy and everything that comes with that. I am choosing to eat this instead of that.'

Focus on maintaining self-discipline by choice instead of thoughts of deprivation.

Accountability

"You must take personal responsibility. You cannot change the circumstances, the seasons, or the wind, but you can change yourself. That is something you have charge of." - Jim Rohn

After your goals are established you will need to set up a system of accountability to do what is required every day to meet your goals. That accountability can be through a friend, family member, or a professional health coach.

You want to share your goals and then regularly discuss your progress and challenges. This sounding board needs to be encouraging to support you when things are tough and to be there to celebrate when you achieve your milestones.

If you have a friend who is also on a quest to achieve health goals, you can work together. Some people have gym or workout partners and the support is reciprocal. Just be sure to pick the right partner. As they say misery loves company and you do not want a codependent type relationship that leads you both to revert to bad habits.

Plan how you will reward yourself and celebrate when you achieve your milestones and goals.

Never stop pursuing optimum health. When you reach a goal have a new one ready to replace your achievement. This will keep you on track for good health and prevent you from falling into any old undesirable habits.

Attitude

"Positive thinking will let you do everything better than negative thinking will." - Zig Ziglar

Attitude is the number one influencer for starting a program of health and fitness and reaching your goals.

- A positive attitude will help you maintain persistence, keep you from giving up, and help you overcome obstacles.
- A positive attitude will help you recognize situations over which you do not have control such as genetics, health issues, age, or history.
- A positive attitude will put these things in perspective and keep them from affecting your progress.

That all sounds great right? But how do you develop and maintain the right attitude?

Focus on the Positive

"The fact is that self-esteem and your circumstances are only indirectly related. There is another intervening factor that determines self-esteem 100 percent of the time: your thoughts." Matthew McKay

You can train your mind to seek out and focus on positive events, situations, and thoughts.

When you develop a steady positive attitude your thoughts will lead you to self-motivation, solutions, feelings of health, confidence, progress, good choices, and creativity.

Your thoughts will move away from self-doubt, blame, mistakes, procrastination, and poor choices.

A positive attitude helps you see your goals are possible and helps you realize them.

Focus on Your 'Why'

Keep your 'why' in focus every day. See each goal as an inevitable event that will happen. Use positive visual techniques such as posting pictures where you will see them each day. These images could be of yourself when you were fit or of other people that are fit.

Remove Negativity

"You are the only one who can control the way you think. Make sure you nourish the positive thoughts and weed out the negative ones!" - Catherine Pulsifer

Your attitude is what dictates how you will react to the obstacles, challenges, and achievements in your life. A negative attitude can make obstacles insurmountable and stop you in your tracks.

Negativity is toxic and can diminish or destroy your chances of reaching your goals. And even if you do achieve a goal, negativity can devalue the importance and seek out reasons to defeat self-confidence.

You need to take control of as much of the input in your life as possible. Avoid negative people and situations. People that complain, blame others, have a victim attitude, put you down, and are not ethical all degrade your attitude and are obstacles between you and your goals. Remove these people from your life or at least severely limit your exposure to them.

The same applies to situations. If you find yourself with a group of people that are allowing themselves to be negatively influenced or are jumping on the negative bandwagon with others that is your sign that the time has come to exit. Negativity is contagious.

You can also practice these same methods with your own thoughts. When you find negative thoughts creeping in, stop and replace them with positive thinking.

Learn to filter your environment by choosing positive people and limiting the input of news and other negative information.

Seek Out Positive Influence
Surround yourself with positive people that will support you in your pursuits. Choose friends that cheer you on and help you succeed. Read positive and inspirational material and books. Listen to positive podcasts and audio books.

Be Grateful

"The way to develop the best that is in a person is by appreciation and encouragement." - Charles Schwab

I like to focus on reasons to be happy. I keep adding to a list of all the things I am grateful for in my life. Creating and reading this list each day motivates me and reinforces a positive upbeat attitude to start the day.

You need to learn what works best for you to create and live with a positive attitude. Then you can set your goals knowing that you can actually reach them.

4. How Does Your Sleep Affect Your Health?

"Sleep is the golden chain that ties health and our bodies together." – Thomas Dekker

Sleep is as important as diet and exercise to maintaining good health for your mind and body.

Getting enough sleep can help you:

- Get sick less often
- Stay at a healthy weight
- Lower your risk for serious health problems, like diabetes and heart disease
- Reduce stress and improve your mood
- Think more clearly and do better in school and at work
- Get along better with people

- Make good decisions and avoid injuries – for example, sleepy drivers cause thousands of car accidents every year

How much sleep do you need?

Most adults need 7 to 8 hours of good quality sleep on a regular schedule each night. Make changes to your routine if you can't find enough time to sleep.

Getting enough sleep isn't only about total hours of sleep. It's also important to get good quality sleep on a regular schedule so you feel rested when you wake up.

If you often have trouble sleeping – or if you often still feel tired after sleeping – talk with your doctor.

Why Does When You Sleep Matter?

Yes. Your body sets your "biological clock" according to the pattern of daylight where you live. This helps you naturally get sleepy at night and stay alert during the day.

Many things can make it harder for you to sleep, including:

- Stress or anxiety
- Pain
- Certain health conditions, like heartburn or asthma
- Some medicines
- Caffeine (usually from coffee, tea, and soda)
- Alcohol and other drugs
- Untreated sleep disorders, like sleep apnea or insomnia

If you are having trouble sleeping, try making changes to your routine to get the sleep you need. You may want to:

- Change what you do during the day – for example, get your physical activity in the morning instead of at night.
- Create a comfortable sleep environment — and make sure your bedroom is dark and quiet.

- Set a bedtime routine – and go to bed at the same time every night.

How can I tell if I have a sleep disorder?

Sleep disorders can cause many different problems. Keep in mind that it's normal to have trouble sleeping every now and then. People with sleep disorders generally experience these problems on a regular basis.

Common signs of sleep disorders include:

- Trouble falling or staying asleep
- Still feeling tired after a good night's sleep
- Sleepiness during the day that makes it difficult to do everyday activities, like driving a car or concentrating at work
- Frequent loud snoring
- Pauses in breathing or gasping while sleeping
- Itchy feelings in your legs or arms at night that feel better when you move or massage the area

- Trouble moving your arms and legs when you wake up

If you have any of these signs, talk to a doctor or nurse. You may need to be tested or treated for a sleep disorder.

Change Your Daytime Habits

Making small changes to your daily routine can help you get the sleep you need.

- Try to spend some time outdoors every day.
- Plan your physical activity for earlier in the day, not right before you go to bed.
- Stay away from caffeine (including coffee, tea, and soda) late in the day.
- If you have trouble sleeping at night, limit daytime naps to 20 minutes or less.
- If you drink alcohol, drink only in moderation. This means no more than 1 drink a day for women and no more than 2 drinks a day for men. Alcohol can keep you from sleeping well.

- Don't eat a big meal close to bedtime.
- Quit smoking. The nicotine in cigarettes can make it harder for you to sleep.
- Change Your Nighttime Habits
- Create a good sleep environment.
- Make sure your bedroom is dark. If there are streetlights near your window, try putting up light-blocking curtains.
- Keep your bedroom quiet.
- Consider keeping electronic devices – like TVs, computers, and smart phones – out of the bedroom.
- Set a bedtime routine.
- Go to bed at the same time every night.
- Get the same amount of sleep each night.
- Avoid eating, talking on the phone, or reading in bed.
- Avoid using computers or smart phones, watching TV, or playing video games at bedtime.

If you find yourself up at night worrying about things, try meditation to relax and reduce stress.

Types of Meditation to Reduce Stress

You can feel healthier and happier by using meditation to reduces stress. The practice triggers your relaxation response—the rest-and-digest part of your nervous system that makes you feel calm and focused.

Our day-to-day lives often put us in fight-or-flight mode. To combat this, use these types of meditation to reduce stress.

What is Mindfulness Meditation?

Mindfulness means paying attention "on purpose, in the present moment, and non-judgmentally."

An informal mindfulness practice might be focusing on eating by paying attention to the taste, texture, smell, look, and even sound of your food.

Formal Mindfulness Meditation to Reduce Stress

A formal mindfulness practice means sitting in meditation to reduce stress. To begin, set a timer for 10 minutes. Make yourself comfortable. You can sit, stand, walk, or lie down. Notice the sensations in your body. Then bring your attention to the breath.

Your mind will wander away from the breath. That's normal. Don't try to stop thinking. Just gently bring your attention back to the breath whenever you notice yourself engage the chatter.

Mantra Meditation to Reduce Stress

Mantra meditation consists of repeating the same phrase or word for a specified amount of time.

To begin, choose the mantra you will use. "Om" is a sacred sound that represents ultimate reality in Hinduism. You can use this popular choice or pick a word, noise, or short sentence that has deep meaning to you.

Then set a timer for 10 minutes. You can sit, stand, walk, or lie down. Take note of your bodily sensation and your breath. Then begin repeating the mantra in your head or out loud. Gently bring your attention back to your chant each time you feel distracted.

Yoga

Yoga is type of exercise and a meditation to reduce stress. The word means "union with the divine" in Sanskrit.

Learn yoga by taking a class, watching a video, or downloading an app. You will be instructed on how to pose in this mind-body meditation to reduce stress. The concentration required forces you to focus on your body and breath instead of your day to day life.

Mindfulness asks you to focus on your breath. Mantra asks you to focus on your chant. Yoga asks you to focus on your body. You can practice meditation to reduce stress by focusing your mind on just one thing instead of overwhelming yourself daily worries.

Keep a sleep diary for a week and share it with your doctor. A doctor can suggest different sleep routines or medicines to treat sleep disorders. Talk with a doctor before trying over-the-counter sleep medicine.

Up at night wondering how to stop insomnia? Most health professionals recommend that adults get 7-9 hours of sleep daily. But getting the sleep you need isn't that simple when you have insomnia, a sleep disorder that makes falling and staying asleep a challenge. While there are medications that can knock you out for the night, they can be habit-forming and have unpleasant side effects. But that doesn't mean you can't kick insomnia to the curb for good.

Here are five of the most trusted remedies for how to stop insomnia:

Wake up at the same time every day. You might just need to train your body to wake and fall asleep at a consistent time. Resist the temptation to sleep in on weekends if you can and try to go to bed around the same time every night.

Say goodbye to caffeine. If you're addicted to your morning cup of Joe, replacing that with something decaffeinated may seem like a scary thought. However, the benefits outweigh any initial fear you may have. Caffeine can stay in the body for hours, playing havoc with your ability to fall asleep. Try to wean yourself off caffeine so you're not reliant on the energy jolt anymore and can fall asleep sooner.

Nix the naps. Although skipping naps might seem counter intuitive when you are tired, catching some shut-eye when you're supposed to be awake can confuse your body. Better to establish a bedtime ritual and stick to your schedule so you don't need a nap.

Address your stress. If worrying consumes you as soon as you hit the pillow, consider addressing the issue before you even enter the bedroom. Maybe do yoga before bed or sit at the kitchen table and plan your next day while saying goodbye to anything that caused stress during the day.

Drink some chamomile tea before bed. Chamomile has been used for hundreds of years as a reliable and safe sleep remedy. Just avoid adding sugar to your tea, since tea acts as a stimulant.

If after you've tried the natural remedies for insomnia, you still find yourself struggling to fall asleep, consider talking to your doctor or a health coach about how to stop insomnia. They may be able to address possible medications or habits that could be affecting your sleep patterns and offer alternative solutions.

5. What is the Commitment Myth?

In addition to this massive disconnect with our food, we are being bombarded with messages about commitment that are false.

Myth: All it takes is commitment.

We have all heard the phrase 'Just do it.' Now a slogan for a major shoe brand, this phrase is meant to get you in motion. But staying in motion or sticking to a health regimen requires much more than merely committing.

Every January the gyms and fitness clubs are packed with people that have declared fitness New Year's resolutions. Other people work out at home. Popular activities include weightlifting, aerobic classes, Pilates, kickboxing, Tae-bo, running, walking, sports such as racquetball, basketball, tennis and others, spin classes, swimming, etc.

Why do people join gyms or commit to working out or exercising?

The top 3 reasons include:

1. To be more attractive.
2. To lose weight.
3. To feel better and have more energy.

Studies show that more than 70 per cent of these New Year resolutions are abandon within six weeks every year.

Why?

While people commit with the best intentions, in a society that desires and expects instant gratification, the progress of exercise or the results come too slow.

Many of these people have not

1. Spent the time preparing their mindset for an exercise routine.
2. Made any adjustments to diet even though their appetites increased due to the activity.

3. Allowed the time required for exercise in their busy schedules.
4. Properly assessed their priorities and other involvements such as work, relationships, children, and old habits take precedence.

Soon the effort required for this physical commitment outweighs their desire for a change. People give up and feel defeated.

So, what can you do to make your health goals happen once and for all?

People that get a good health coach more than double their chances of making their New Year's health resolutions stick.

Why?

A good health coach will help you analyze what you need to be doing, help you develop a plan, and support and motivate you to do what it takes to get where you want to be.

What do professional athletes all have in common? They have coaches. While you might not aspire to be a professional athlete, the same monitoring, support and encouragement can be yours with a great health coach. That's what you need to greatly increase your potential of achieving your goals.

Imagine being at your ideal weight, feeling terrific and having all the energy you need from sun up to when your head hits the pillow and then sleeping soundly through the night. How much more could you accomplish and how better could you relax?

My coaching philosophy is behavior based. This is simple: if you want different results you will need to take different actions and make them habits. My job is to help you determine the exact actions for your situation and goals and help you develop the habits that will get you where you want to be and keep you there.

If you are not satisfied with your state of fitness; what you have been doing to get where you are will not get you where you want to be.

Without changing behaviors, you will predictably fail to reach your goals.

Steady motivation, however, guides you through all of the difficulties of achieving fitness and continues to energize your efforts to maintain your fitness even after you have reached your initial goals. When considering why you want to be fit, wanting to look good is a natural desire, but is best considered as a secondary motivation or as a side effect of your fitness efforts. The best and most effective motivation is achieving health.

You only have one body, and without the health of that body, you cannot fully experience your life. Even if occasional back pain, low energy levels, or high cholesterol do not seem to be holding you back now, the health of your body directly influences how quickly your body ages and how limiting your body will be in that old age. We all know or have seen a seventy-year-old who is still in amazingly good health and continues to live life to the fullest, but much more common are people even in their fifties who suffer severe limitations to their abilities to enjoy and experience life because of the poor condition of their bodies.

Your goal for achieving fitness should be to live to be a ripe old age and to enjoy every minute of life. Perhaps you have children or grandchildren who you want to be able to play with and watch mature. Maybe you enjoy traveling or playing sports and don't want to have to give up the things you love because of physical limitations that could have been prevented.

When you are fit, your biological age is lower, your physical limitations are less, and your chances of suffering from diseases and injuries are reduced. If health is you goal, you will inevitably achieve good looks as well, but, more importantly, you will give your body the treatment and attention needed to ensure you have the best vehicle for life possible.

6. What is the Best Exercise for You?

"The higher your energy level, the more efficient your body. The more efficient your body, the better you feel and the more you will use your talent to produce outstanding results." - Tony Robbins

Visit your physician before starting and exercise program and determining what exercises are best for you.

How Can You Have Enough Workout Energy?

Ask yourself these three questions about your workout energy:

- Do you ever get tired during your workouts, while running or playing sports?
- Do you feel your performance is sometimes falling short?
- Maybe you have enough workout or game energy but what about afterwards: are

you tired longer than you think you should be during recovery?

If you answered 'yes' to any of these questions, I can help. What's happening with your energy when you work out or compete in sports? When you work out, run, or play competitive sports your body uses your 'energy inventory'. This energy inventory is glycogen that is stored mostly in your liver and skeletal muscles. Glycogen stored in your muscle is ready to fuel your muscles. Glycogen in your liver is used throughout your body though the two other big users are your brain and spinal cord.

As you work out or compete, your body is converting the glycogen stored into energy. If your energy levels are not sufficient, your performance and recovery will suffer keeping you from doing your best.

The body inventories about 2,000 calories of glucose as glycogen. This can limit athletic performance when you can burn that number of calories in just a couple of hours. When you run out of glycogen, performing becomes a challenge. This experience is sometimes referred to as 'hitting a wall'.

How can you help ensure your glycogen storage levels are enough for your workout energy activities and have what you need for quick recovery?

How much glycogen inventory your body has built up in these cells depends on your activities, amount of rest, and how you are fueling your body (what you eat).

How can you be READY? Here are my tips for having enough workout energy:

<u>READY</u>
R-Rest
E-Eat
A-Aerobics
D-Drink
Y-Yardstick

Rest

Getting enough rest is imperative for workout energy. Everyone is unique and only you know the right amount of sleep and rest for your optimum energy levels.

Eat

Eat well and eat consistently. If you normally eat four or five small meals a day do so every day. Skipping meals, mixing up the times or not choosing the right foods will wreak havoc with your energy levels. If you don't like heavy meals, east smaller ones.

Foods that will supply your energy include fruits, nuts, oats, fruits, green vegetables, and others. Complex carbohydrates increase glycogen enabling your body to be prepared for workouts and competition. Refined carbs such as sugar cereals, white bread, and processed foods give you a boost but cause a crash and fatigue soon after.

Take energy snacks on the go such as crackers and cheese, nuts, legumes, protein bars, or yogurt. If you are unsure of what foods work best for your daily activities, our coaching program will evaluate your needs.

There is a dizzying quantity of energy boosting supplements on the market. Some of these supplements can improve and increase your energy levels. Avoid the drinks and supplements that are filled with sugar caffeine. The energy is short lived, and they have been linked to negative side effects.

Aerobics Workouts

Start your day and your workouts by giving your heart and circulation some exercise. A pre-workout are aerobic activities that kickstart your muscles within minutes These exercises include jogging, brisk walking, or dancing.

Drink

Drink fluids such as pure drinking water to stay hydrated. Dehydrating can cause sudden fatigue. Your body loses water through perspiration. 10 ounces of water every 10 to 15 minutes of exercise is recommended. Sports beverages do contain carbs and potassium, though these drinks are intended for longer endurance activities.

Yardstick

Yardstick or monitor your body so that you are getting the right amounts of rest, food, exercise and fluids. Our coaching program helps you measure your results so that you can make informed choices. Measuring also helps you see where you can improve and keeps you motivated. Find out how our coaching program helps you track your energy levels and workout results.

Note: Glycogen is should not be confused with the hormone glucagon, which is also important in carbohydrate metabolism and blood glucose control.

Home Workouts You Can Do with No Equipment

Home workouts are becoming more popular. The mass exodus from gyms is being brought on by a few factors. Gyms are expensive. They are inconvenient. You have to drive to and from the gym, wasting precious time. Many people are choosing to use what nature gave us: the outdoors and our own bodies.

If you are choosing to do home workouts, here are a few of the best no-equipment exercises you can perform at home, in the park, or where ever else you find yourself.

King of the Home Workout: Squat

Squatting is a basic human movement. Known as the "King of Exercises," most of the muscle groups in your body will get engaged when you perform a squat. Your core and large lower muscles will get the biggest hit.

To do a basic squat, stand straight with your knees at hips-width distance apart. Lower down as if you are going to sit, keeping your heels on the ground, your back straight, and your toes behind your knees. Once you are at your max, straighten your legs, pushing off through your heels and the balls of your feet.

This home workout has infinite variability. From the partial squat for the extreme beginner to the pistol squat for the very advanced, this move should remain in your arsenal no matter your fitness level.

Core Home Workout: Plank

The plank is another exercise that is very core intensive but hits other parts of your body including your glutes and hamstrings. Some iterations can also strengthen your shoulder and arms.

To perform a basic forearm plank, get in the same position as you would for a push-up but rest your forearms on the floor and position your elbows beneath your shoulders. Keep your back in a straight line from heel to head and keep your back parallel to the floor. Hold the position as long as you can.

Once you've mastered this home workout, you can advance to side planks, caterpillar planks, and plank jacks.

Upper Body Home Workout: Push-Ups

This popular exercise is well-known for a reason. The push up works your chest muscles, your shoulders, and your arms. They are a fast and effective way to build strength in your upper body.

To do a proper push-up, get into position with your hands slightly further apart than your shoulders. Make sure that your body is a straight line from heel to head and that your feet are at a comfortable distance apart. Slowly lower yourself down, bending your elbows back to a 90-degree angle until your chest just about touches the floor, and then raise yourself back up until your arms are completely straight.

More challenging variations include the clap push-up, grasshopper push-up, and dive bomber push-up.

Doing these three home workouts will build your strength and endurance without you having to fork over cash to anyone.

Strength Training

Strength training can be defined as an exercise designed to improve muscle strength, increase lean muscle mass, maintain bone density, decrease excess body fat (by increasing muscle metabolism), improve balance, reduce joint pain and ultimately provide additional psychological benefits. In fact, there are so many health, fitness and mental well-being advantages associated with regularly performing a strength training routine that is an important part of all fitness practices.

A strength exercise is an activity that makes your muscles work harder than with typical activity. By increasing your muscles' strength, size, power and endurance (stamina), you will help your body handle daily activities and other strenuous activities with more ease. These activities involve using your body weight or working against a resistance. For your body to benefit the most from strengthening exercises, you should try to do two or more sessions of muscle strengthening exercises a week.

Some examples of muscle-strengthening activities include, but are not limited to:

- lifting weights (free weights or plated machines)
- working with resistance bands
- climbing stairs
- hill walking
- cycling
- dance

- push-ups, sit-ups and squats (body weight exercises)
- Yoga
- Pilates

As noted above, the term "strength training" can be used to describe an exercise type that is designed to improve muscular strength and endurance. All exercise types that promote increases in muscular strength and lean muscle tissue can further be defined as resistance training. Resistance training can then be defined as performing an exercise that forces the muscles to contract (shorten) when moving an object of weight.

First, it's important to define "functional training". The term functional training is meant to describe exercises and programming that makes you better at a task. This ranges from sports performance to activities of daily living.

If an exercise makes life a little easier for you, or makes you a better athlete, the exercise can be considered functional. It's also important to understand that strength and power (ability to generate force quickly) improves function and performance. You cannot achieve a high rate of power without first being relatively strong.

BODY WEIGHT EXERCISES: Bodyweight training utilizes movements such as pushing, pulling, squatting, bending, twisting and balancing. The term is simple where you use your own body's weight for resistance against gravity. It is recognized that bodyweight exercises can increase strength, power, endurance, speed, flexibility, coordination and balance.

CORE TRAINING: The area of the body, which is commonly referred to as the core, is your midsection and it involves all your muscles in that area including the front, back and sides. These foundation muscles work as stabilizers for the entire body and keeping these core muscles strong will help with your posture and help create a solid base for your body, allowing you to stay upright and stand strong on your two feet. While core work does help produce toned abdominal muscles, core exercises include a lot more than just crunches.

Functional core training is about power, strength and stabilization. Challenging your core not only improves balance and functional movement, it also provides support for daily tasks and creates that toned look that so many people dream about. Activation of these muscles is possible by recruiting the right fibers in the movement. One of the most used core exercises is the plank. It is an isometric contraction, but the muscles are working. Try regular and side planks to increase your core strength first before working on harder core exercises. Training the core muscles will help prevent injuries and be the foundation of good mechanics while working or exercising properly.

Weight Machines and Free Weights

Free Weights include dumbbells, barbells, kettlebells, and anything else you can pick up and hold. They promote your body to work against gravity while moving the weight. Some exercises may require use of a bench to sit or lie on, or other equipment such as a squat cage to help you safely work with the weight. Dumbbell exercises allow coordination of several different muscles to work together to produce and stabilize joint motion. Using lighter dumbbells multiplane movement patterns improves coordination between multiple muscles activated in this pattern. Using heavier dumbbells can increase the number of muscle fibers activated within a specific muscle.

Machines include anything that you sit in, or on, while you pull or push a lever through a specific range of motion. Machines are grounded and typically provide more support while isolating a muscle group in a particular plane. For example, a leg extension machine or a chest press machine has a pulley that lifts a stack of weights that you have selected to lift by putting a pin in the proper space. Cable machines have characteristics of both. To use a cable machine, you pull on a handle attached to a cord—the cable—which in turn lifts the weights from a stack. Although they are a type of machine, they do not limit use in an isolated plane of motion. That means cable machine exercises have a lot in common with free weight exercises.

Circuit Training

The main foundation of circuit training is to increase muscle strength, endurance, flexibility and coordination during a variety of high- intensity exercises. Each training session usually includes a combination of both aerobic exercise and strength training. However, circuit training can include whatever type of exercise you want, in whatever combination helps you accomplish your exercise goals. This could mean your circuit training routine includes only aerobics or only strength training. Although it may look a bit confusing to an observer, there is method to the craziness that compliments this intense form of exercise. Its pace can give you an awesome cardiovascular workout because you can adapt the exercises to your current level of fitness. An exercise circuit is one completion of all prescribed exercises in the program, accomplishing about 10-25 reps at each station, lasting between 30 seconds and 3 minutes, and then move on to the next station. Seeing that circuit training is a total body workout, you are less likely to get bored during the workouts.

Muscle Power Training

Muscle power is the relationship between strength and power and demonstrates how much force a muscle can exhibit and how quickly the force can be produced. When training for power, quality of movement is more important than quantity of repetitions. Performing short sets with maximal intensity combined with rests that are long enough for you to work at maximum intensity during each set will help you to develop more power. Power is intimately related to force and time, which can be expressed in the simple formula:

Traditional strength training typically alters the top half of this equation – increasing the ability to apply a maximum amount of force. But for power to be maximized the time component must also be altered.

Some examples of power activities include, but are not limited to:

- Long jumps
- Medicine ball overhead throws
- clapping push-ups
- Plyometrics
- jump squats

Cardiovascular Conditioning (CV)

Cardio exercise is any exercise that raises your heart rate and respiration while using large muscle groups repetitively and rhythmically. Your heart is a muscle, so it needs to be worked for it to become stronger. This movement makes your heart stronger and a stronger heart makes for a more efficient and healthy body. When you do a cardio session, you're giving your heart, lungs and circulatory system, as well as any other muscle groups that you use, a good workout. Cardio exercise is extremely important because a stronger cardio-vascular system means more capillaries (very small blood vessels that transport blood and oxygen to the working skeletal muscle) deliver more oxygen and nutrients to the cells in your muscles. Cardio exercise uses large muscle movement over a sustained period of time keeping your heart rate elevated.

Max Heart Rate: It is recommended that you exercise within 55 to 85 percent of your maximum heart rate (MHR) for at least 20 to 30 minutes to get the best results from aerobic exercise. The Max Heart Rate (roughly calculated as 220 minus your age) is the upper limit of what your cardiovascular system can handle during physical activity. Example: 220-50 = 170 beats per minute (bpm) x .55-.85 (93.5 bpm- 144.5 bpm)

Before starting any new exercise program, it is important to know if you are healthy enough to increase your activity level. Please check with a health care professional on any limitations or restrictions you may have, particularly if you have a chronic health condition.

American Heart Association Recommendation

For Overall Cardiovascular Health: At least 30 minutes of moderate-intensity aerobic activity at least 5 days per week. Moderate- to high-intensity muscle-strengthening activity at least 2 days per week for additional health benefits.

For Lowering Blood Pressure and Cholesterol

An average 40 minutes of moderate- to vigorous-intensity aerobic activity 3 or 4 times per week.

There are many different types of CV exercise. The most effective are exercises that use the largest muscle groups in the body and require you to support your own bodyweight while exercising. Walking, jogging and running, while excellent fat burning exercise, are excellent for your CV workout because they use the large muscles of the legs and you have to weight bear throughout your workout.

Not only is a CV workout healthy for your heart and lungs, there are many other benefits of cardio exercise. Weight loss lowers blood pressure and cholesterol, increased bone density, reduces stress & depression, better sleep, maintain muscle strength into old age, more energy, live longer, and less likely to get sick.

Some of the Best Cardio Workouts Are:

Walking: This is the easiest and safest way to start getting in your cardio.

Elliptical: Minimal impact on the knees and hips but calorie burning is still high. When you increase the incline, you will activate more muscles.

Running: Distance or sprints? Steading running burns calories, but sprints take it to the next level.

High Intensity Interval Training (HIIT): Short intervals at maximum intensity followed by short periods of rest. More efficient great cardio workout in just 20 or 30 minutes, increases endurance more quickly burning more calories, and adds variety, reducing boredom.

Bike Riding or Cycling: Cycling uses large muscle groups in the legs and helps elevate your heart rate. Can do it inside or outside.

Stair Climber: Uses more muscles than walking.

Jumping Rope: Cheap, easy and burns tons of calories

Swimming: This is a total body workout even while treading water. Swimming laps is best and changing up the strokes allows you to use different muscles while the continuous pace works your heart and lungs.

Rowing: Works both the upper and lower body and is low stress on joints and ligaments.

Circuit Training: When you work out at a high intensity the blood starts to pump a lot harder and that challenges the heart.

Dance: continuous movement while weight bearing using arms and exaggerated hip movements. Zumba or any other form has benefits.

Weight Loss with Cardio

Is a cardio or strength-training workout better for weight loss?

In a nut shell, weight loss happens when you burn more calories than you eat. While some people prefer to cut calories through their diets, it helps to have a combination of things: cardio, strength training, and a healthy low-calorie diet.

Strength training builds lean muscle mass, which both increases your metabolism and decreases fat. So, the more muscle you build, the more calories you burn on a day-to-day basis.

Should you start with cardio or strength training? If you're hitting the treadmill for an intense cardio session and then plan to hit the weights afterward, you'll have little left in your tank to make your resistance training count. When it comes to doing a full, high-intensity cardio session and an entire resistance training workout, perform each on separate days so you can give each one your all and burn more calories in the process.

Researchers crunched the numbers of people who did different workouts, each of which was sequenced in a different way, and found that if you want more bang for your workout buck, it's best to perform cardio before resistance training. Why does cardio come in at No. 1? It first allows you to perform at your desired intensity while lessening your chances of unknowingly training at too high of an intensity, which could result in injury.

Not only does muscle burn calories and allows you to lose weight, it also helps with your cardio routines. As an example, having strong glutes for running helps you go faster for longer, which burns more calories. And doing exercises to strengthen your core can help you maintain form for biking, which can also help you burn more calories.

High-Intensity Interval Training Basics

High-Intensity Interval Training alternates short bursts of pushing your body to its limits (70%-90% of your maximum heart rate) with shorter rest periods (60%-65% of your maximum heart rate). There isn't a standard amount of time for the intervals. One program might have you work out 55 seconds and rest 5 seconds, while another has you work out 5 minutes and rest 1 minute.

How to handle your rest period also isn't a prescribed. Some practitioners believe in complete stillness, while others think that low-intensity exercise like walking or stretching optimizes your routine. Keep in mind that your "intense" is not the same as the next persons. If you can speak during the more active phase of your workout, you need to ramp it up.

High-Intensity Interval Training distinguishes itself from weight lifting and steady state cardio by how often you can train. While steady state cardio and weight training can be done safely every day, HIIT should only be practiced a maximum of three times per week.

Pros of High-Intensity Interval Training

Due to the intensity of the training, this exercise paradigm demands only about 30 minutes of your time per work out, as opposed to the 60 minutes or more than a gentler exercise routine would ask of you.

In those 30 minutes, you are going to burn a lot of calories. You burn 9-13 calories per minute in a HIIT workout. Compare this to weight lifting and cardio, both of which burn about 1.5-3 calories per minute.

One of the greatest benefits that you'll get from HIIT is that the practice will increase your VO2 max. This is how much oxygen your body is capable of consuming and a general health indicator.

High-Intensity Interval Training HIIT at Home

HIIT is any exercise done with enough intensity and can be done anywhere. You don't need to go to the gym or to buy any equipment. Your body weight is more than enough to build muscle doing jumping jacks, push-ups, or squats.

Cons of High-Intensity Interval Training

As the name indicates, these are intense workouts. If you feel extremely uncomfortable while exercising, you may be unlikely to continue. You also may increase your risk of injury if you do not train slowly and progressively. You need to be particularly careful about your joints and ligaments when beginning a HIIT regime. While HIIT can be demanding, you get a lot of bang for your buck.

Workout Recovery

We need to make sure our bodies get the right fuel in order to have the best workout recovery. During a workout, we deplete our muscles of glycogen and protein. Without these nutrients, your body is unable to rebound and build muscles.

Give your body a push in the right direction by getting some of these vitamins, foods, and drinks 20 to 45 minutes after a workout.

Vitamins for Workout Recovery

Vitamin D

Myostatin is a protein that inhibits muscle cell growth. Vitamin D decreases the amount of myostatin in your blood, allowing your body to build new cells and tissues.

Vitamin C

Popularly used to help treat the common cold, vitamin C helps your body recover from any metabolic stress by reducing free radicals.

Your body uses vitamin C to produce collagen, which is necessary to build and repair connective tissue during workout recovery.

Vitamin B

Consisting of eight vitamins that are grouped together due to similarities, these micronutrients help your body build cells, metabolize proteins and carbohydrates, and repair muscle.

Food for Workout Recovery

Protein Sources

Branched-Chain Amino Acids (BCAA)

These compounds synthesize protein themselves and support your cells in synthesizing protein. They also slow protein breakdown. These two functions lower your chances of entering into a catabolic crisis, which would worsen your workout recovery.

Eggs

This high protein food is BCAA-rich. Growth-supporting vitamin B12, B6, and iron are present in the yolk.

Yogurt

Unsweetened yogurt provides your body with the high-quality carbohydrates and proteins needed for a great workout recovery. Yogurt also has calcium which builds bones.

Salmon. The omega 3s in fatty fish lower prostaglandins in the blood, a compound that causes inflammation. Inflammation is one of the main causes of discomfort during workout recovery.

Carbohydrate Sources

Sweet potato

This tuber is rich in complex carbs, nutritionally dense, and contains antioxidants and potassium to help your body's workout recovery.

Dark, leafy greens

Kale, swiss chard, and spinach will help reduce inflammation, counteracting the natural stiffness and soreness of a body recovering from stress.

Fluids

Water

Your body loses water through sweat. Dehydration slows your metabolism. Drink water before, during, and after exercise for the best rejuvenation.

Tart Cherry Juice

The nutrients in this drink aid muscle recovery, reduce free radicals in the blood, and decrease muscle damage and strength loss.

Milk

Full of casein, whey, BCAA, carbs, calcium, water, electrolytes and nutrients, milk may be the perfect post-workout meal.

Conclusion

Humans are unique. Each of us is a one of a kind exclusive. Your lifestyle, body, history, genetics, and goals are all distinctive to you.

Mission Zest was founded with a passion and philosophy of serving people from all walks of life. Each wellness coaching session is focused on intently listening to the unique needs of each individual and aligning an optimal nutrition and health program strategy.

Rather than a generic approach, each session is guided through evidence-based practice, expertise and experience across the health, wellness and fitness fields.

If any of the information in this book can benefit you to get healthier, reach your fitness goals, and live longer, I have succeeded. I certainly hope that is the case.

If you found something useful here or have a question or comment, please reach out to me.

About the Author

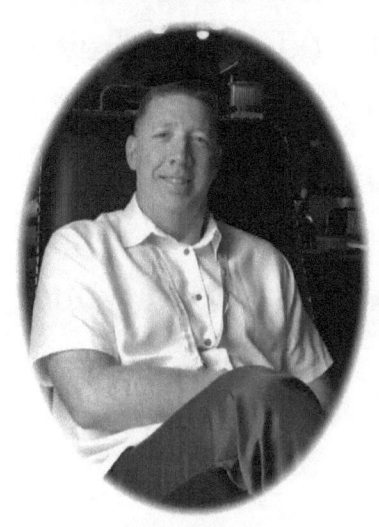

Bob competed successfully in team sports at the high school and collegiate levels. Bob describes his experience, "Being a competitive athlete has taught me a lot about facing adversity, the importance of collaboration and a commitment to constant self-improvement. Spanning a career of eighteen years, I carried these values with me in the business arena providing management leadership, coaching and mentoring for many individuals."

In 2007, Bob and his wife pursued their passion, dream and vision by opening Team Fitness and CrossFit situated in Franklin, MA. As owner operators, this transition enabled them to positively impact the health of thousands of people and truly experience the health, wellness and nutrition industry "live". After a successful sale of the business, they are now engaged with Mission Zest continuing their focus on helping people from all walks of life.

"I would be honored to do the same for you," Bob Flynn.

Contact Information

Mission Zest
Bob Flynn
www.MissionZest.com

Contact Page

http://www.missionzest.com/about/

Facebook:
https://www.facebook.com/MissionZest/

Thank you and all the best,

Bob Flynn
P.N. Certified Health Coach